Fade Pigmentation Naturally

Skin Whitening Techniques To Clear Your complexion. Treat Hyper and Hypopigmentation, Eliminate Blemishes, Dark And Brown Spots, Freckles, Melasma And Age Spots From All Skin Colors At Any Age.

By Ori Laor

Disclaimer

The methods described within this eBook are the author's personal thoughts. They are not intended to be a definitive set of instructions for this project. You may discover there are other methods and materials to accomplish the same end result.

This book is not intended to be a substitute for the medical advice of a licensed physician. The reader should consult with their doctor in any matters relating to his/her health.

Before beginning any new exercise program, it is recommended that you seek medical advice from your personal physician.

The information contained within this eBook is strictly for educational purposes. If you wish to apply ideas contained in this eBook, you are taking full responsibility for your actions.

The author has made every effort to ensure the accuracy of the information within this book was correct at time of publication. The author does not assume and hereby disclaims any liability to any party for any loss, damage, or disruption caused by errors or omissions, whether such errors or omissions result from accident, negligence, or any other cause.

Thank you very much
Ori Laor

Table of Contents

Personal Introduction

Thank you for downloading this fantastic guide - "FADE PIGMENTATION NATURALLY -Skin Whitening Techniques To Clear Your Completion. Treat Hyperpigmentation, Eliminate Blemishes, Dark And Brown Spots, Freckles, Melasma And Age Spots From All Skin Colors At Any Age." I have cleared pigmentation from my face myself and learned over the years all it takes to treat stubborn pigmentation from people of all ages and skin colors efficiently and naturally.

Pigmentation occurs when there is too little or too much of melanin produced by your skin. The skin will either appear dark or discolored due to the melanin secretion. The root cause of the pigmentation is due to the internal factors of the body like hormones and pregnancy. External factors like burning, chemicals, ultraviolet rays, stress and dietary issues also cause skin pigmentation.

Almost everyone has Pigmentation! people who live in a sunny place have pigmentation from early age, Doctors and nurses in hospitals get pigmentation over the years from exposure to the neon lights, people who take or took drugs like birth control pills and antibiotics tend to develop pigmentation and regular mix of genes between people who give birth create in the future pigmentation problems.

Whatever your age, there are few of us who haven't experienced some sort of skin blemish, color change or 'pigmentation'. From sunburn to hormonal changes, Acne and infections – skin color changes can sometimes make us feel self-conscious, worried and searching for answers.

As a professional Aesthetician, I read and research medical books and I have tried to create an easy-to-digest ebook that will help you understand what causes these skin alterations and how you can treat them. I hope it helps.

In This book, I will take your hand and guide you throw everything you need to do to clear your pigmentation problem fast and efficient. I will help you achieve efficiently and naturally the most important steps to make your face clear of melanin and how to always feel and look your best.

For my new Kindle readers, I offer a Free Voucher Gift of 20$. You can find a keyword at the end of this book. Please send it to my mail orilaor@outlook.com, and you will receive a discount for any porches you make for yourself, a member of your family or a friend in LAOR website www.laorcare.com.

About Me

I have a passion for Beauty, Skincare, Anti-aging and well-being methods. In my extensive exploration around the world, I gathered sacred pieces of information that helped me and then other people from all walks of life to look and feel younger. I hold a BA in Art and diplomas for Makeup Artist, Para Medical Aesthetician, Aromatherapy, Naturopathy, and Nutrition consultant. I am a well-known name in T.V scene and in the cosmetic industry, including treating many celebrities. When I was 30 years old, I quit working for others and founded LAOR, a House of natural Beauty and Professional Skin Care and treatments for the face, Body, and Mind.

Since an early age, I suffered from my skin and was carried away with Skincare research, science and well-being. I worked in beauty and style departments in New York and Tel Aviv, based on my experience I invented a revolutionary practice for treating the skin from within – **The Layer system**, Complied with a line of professional cosmetic products and treatments for the face to treat any skin problem.

Ientered the natural cosmetics world with a unique world-view and with one simple, honest purpose: to create a different kind of cosmetic that is Natural and effective. My desire is that each product would provide each with the essence of beauty, based on effective ingredients.

Now, for the past Two Decades, I am designing the products that Men and women across the world love, helping them to look and feel younger with all the secrets of skin care. When I am not working, I love to design and create, read, write and paint. My quest is to bring more beauty to the world and raise self-awareness.

Let's Get Started!

<u>Chapter 1</u>

Pigmentation Source

Skin color is determined by a pigment (melanin) made by specialised cells in the skin (melanocytes). The amount and type of melanin determines a person's skin color – or skin pigmentation. Pigmentation is the colouring of a person's skin. When a person is healthy, his or her skin will appear normal in color. In the case of illness or injury, the person's skin may change color, becoming darker (hyperpigmentation) or lighter (hypopigmentation) Furthermore Patches of discoloration found on your skin are generally considered pigmentation. They're mainly caused by high exposure to the sun and harmful UVA rays. UVA rays will stimulate production of melanin, which is what causes you to tan. The more melanin, the darker your skin looks. Pigmentation usually takes 1-2 decades to form, so prevention from a young age is crucial in stopping Pigmentation from forming.

Pigmentation Types

If you have pigmentation, determine which type you have by referring to these seven most common types.

Freckles

- ✓ Freckles are flat, tanned, and found in the size of matchstick heads.

- ✓ It is caused by uneven distribution of melanin; as a result freckles usually appear uniform in color.

- ✓ Freckles are genetic and usually occur during young age.

Melasma/ Chloasma

- ✓ Melasma is also known as the 'mask of pregnancy,' and commonly occurs to women during their reproduction period.

- ✓ It usually affects females because of the presence of female hormones such as estrogen, progesterone and melanocytes stimulating hormone.

- ✓ Only 1/20 men are affected.

✓ There are three types of melasma: epidermal, dermal and mixed.

Age Spots/Liver Spots

✓ Age spots tend to develop after the age of 40, to which it indicates that the skin has entered its aging period.

✓ When skin ages and is further exposed to environmental damages, melanocytes consistently produce melanin to protect the skin.

✓ Post-Inflammatory Hyperpigmentation (PIH)

PIH develops through inflamed wounds.

✓ When a wound causes skin inflammation, keratinocytes will produce melanin excessively resulting in skin discoloration on the wounded area.

✓ PIH's condition may be aggravated by chemical peels, laser treatments and IPL.

✓ Post-Acne Pigmentation (PAP)

✓ PAP develops from acne lesions that have healed.

✓ It is caused by the overproduction of melanin in reaction to inflammation on the affected area.

Sun Burn Pigmentation (Solar Lentigines) (SBP)

- ✓ SBP develops from the overexposure of sun or ultraviolet sources.

- ✓ SBP is found on areas of the skin that are more exposed to sun or UV damages.

- ✓ Computer Radiation Spots (CRS)

- ✓ CRS develops from extended period of exposure towards computer or mobile phone radiation.

- ✓ Computer and mobile produce static electricity and radiation that damages the skin.

Hypopigmentation

- ✓ Hypopigmentation, which is the absence of normal amounts of melanin (the chemical that gives skin its colour), is almost as common.

- ✓ **This type of pigmentation** – usually caused by disease, injury, burns or other trauma to the skin is trickier to treat then its skin-darkening cousin. Improperly administered skinresurfacing treatments, such as Photofacials, laser peels, or chemical peels can also cause skin damage that result in hypopigmentation.

Hypopigmentation Causes- Some chronic skin disorders can also cause hypopigmentation, such as the following:

- ✓ **Albinism** - characterised by colourless skin, hair, and eyes that occurs because skin cells produce little or no melanin.

- ✓ **Vitiligo** - characterized by patchy loss of skin colour that occurs when skin cells that produce melanin die or stop production for no known reason.

- ✓ **Seborrheic dermatitis** - an inflammatory skin disease characterised by red, scaly, itchy patches of skin in areas prone to oiliness.

- ✓ **Tinea versicolor** – This is caused by fungal (yeast) infection and characterised by scaly, itchy patches of lighter or pinkish skin.

- ✓ **Pityriasis alba** - most commonly affects children and is characterised by colourless, scaly skin patches.

- ✓ **Post-inflammatory hypopigmentation (PIH)** - In situations where hypopigmentation is the result of skin inflammation or damage, the condition may be referred to as post-inflammatory hypopigmentation, or PIH. This can get confusing because PIH is also used to refer to post-inflammatory hyperpigmentation, a skin condition where pigmentation is increased, not decreased.

Treatment Methods

Some skin pigmentation is inevitable in harsh desert climate. Whether your pigmentation is sun induced or a result of hormonal activity (Melasma), genetics or trauma to the skin, it ages your appearance and can erode your confidence.

The skin consists of two main layers; the epidermis which is the upper layer and the dermis which is the lower layer. Within, the lowest layer of the epidermis, are cells called melanocytes, which are responsible for producing the pigment called melanin. This melanin production is what gives our skin its genetically predetermined color and when overstimulated, can produce excess pigmentation.

While we all know the telltale signs of spending too much time in the sun, hormonal pigmentation, or Melasma, is less commonly recognized. Melasma is characterized by patchy brown discolouration of the skin, commonly seen on the cheeks, chin, forehead and upper lip in a symmetrical pattern. It primarily occurs in women but can also appear in men. While it can affect all racial and ethnic groups it is more common in darker skinned individuals.

Treating pigmentation of any kind in the skin can be complicated and there are many options. Often using a combination of technologies yields better, longer lasting results and this is why it pays to go to a professional with access to multiple technologies. One laser doesn't fix all in this case! Melasma, being hormonally stimulated, is particularly difficult to treat as too aggressive or inappropriate treatment can often exacerbate the condition.

Some of the more common treatments for pigmentation include:

- ✓ Professional Procedures

- ✓ Medical Grade Skin Care Products

- ✓ Cosmetic Peels and Aesthetic Treatments

IPL Intense Pulsed Light is a quick, effective and straightforward treatment, with no downtime, that helps fade the brown patches giving the skin a more even, 'cleaner' appearance within a few days. Usually, only 2-3 treatments are required at 2-4 week intervals. Any area affected can be treated and these are most commonly the face, neck, décolletage, hands/arms and back.

For pigment that is more stubborn or deeper in the skin, fractionated lasers are very effective. Fractionated lasers treat a fraction of the skin at a time while leaving surrounding healthy skin intact, delivering remarkable improvement with minimal downtime. This medical procedure lightens pigmentation with the added benefit of pore refinement, resurfacing of the skin as well as the stimulation of collagen. It can be used to treat Melasma and for prematurely aged, sun damaged skin, it is fantastic.

Various masks and peels and creams containing lightening agents can be used either to maintain the results of light based technologies, or as a slower but gentler approach to pigmentation. Whenever treating pigmentation of any cause, it is absolutely essential the home care regime contains medical grade cosmecuticals that have been individualized to your skins needs. over the counter product will simply be wasting your time and money. Antioxidants like vitamins A, B3 and C, Retinol as well as Alpha and Beta Hydroxyl acids work synergistically to fade pigmentation, calm melanocyte activity, stimulate collagen and boost the skins natural immunity.

Treating pigmentation isn't just about fading what is on the surface. It is also about restoring health and balance to the skin. Isn't that what we all want? Of course, any skincare regime in every part of the world must include an minimum 30 SPF sunscreen. While most of us hate wearing them, there are new sun block creams that are light and quickly absorbed. You may even be able to get your children to wear it!

If you do suffer from pigmentation, be reassured there is help available, but choose wisely where you go to get that help. Inappropriate or too aggressive treatment can be disastrous but with the correct treatment approach and the guidance of experienced Aestheticians, you can regain control of your skin and start to get your confidence back.

With Melasma, the melanocytes become over stimulated and over produce melanin in response to changes in oestrogen and progesterone levels. This melanin becomes trapped in the epidermis and may also extend to the dermis, making it difficult to treat. Pigmented cells then slowly migrate to the surface, making the pigmentation visible. The most common cause is pregnancy or oral contraceptive use but it can occur for no apparent reason.

While few abnormalities in skin color, like albinism, cannot be treated, other types of skin pigmentation can be treated to varying degrees depending on the cause and the severity.

Freckles is a very common type of skin pigmentation mostly faced by Caucasians. The concentrated clusters of melanin become worse with exposure to sunlight. So first These can be treated with sun block creams and these days, professional pigmentation treatmentswith safe creams are done to remove them efficiently, and I will go through all the ingredients later in this book.

Laser pigmentation removal is also used to treat age spots that occur due to old age. Skin whitening creams and anti-aging creams and lotions also help minimize and control age or liver spots. Aesthetic clinics employs the latest advanced techniques to lighten the skin's color. Highly experienced aesthetician can bring about long-lasting results.

Production of extra melanin leads to hyperpigmentation. Medications and skin bleaching creams prescribed by an aesthetic doctor are as effective as laser treatment. Laser treatment is only ideal for small patches and not for wide spread discoloration.

Birthmarks are normally brown, black or blue in color. They are flat, and you can undergo laser treatment to reduce their appearance. Laser treatment will make them lighter and less visible. Sometimes, melasma appears in women during pregnancy and fades away after birth; prescription and Professional creams are enough to treat it.

Port-wine stains and hemangioma are two other types of skin pigmentation that can be treated with creams and laser treatment or cosmetic peels. Cosmetic peels are highly effective in treating a range of skin pigmentation disorders. There can be significant change after the first peel. The recommended number of peels has an excellent effect in treating skin damage due to sun exposure or aging.

IPL - Advanced Intense Pulsed Light technology methods have a greater degree of penetration, they are precise and help target more intense and severe discoloration when compared to chemical peels and microdermabrasion. IPL treatment removes discoloration by breaking down the skin. After a few days, the darkened tissues fall off. There is some discomfort after the procedure, and creams need to be applied to reduce pain and irritation. It is wise to use professional lightening creams when the skin heals to keep the skin clear For long-lasting results.

Hypopigmentation Treatments

- ✓ Hypopigmentation treatment options are often limited. Treating post-inflammatory hypopigmentation may involve the use of topical corticosteroids or tars (topical cream), light or laser treatment, or surgical skin grafting. Although the numerous lasers and other light-based treatments available today are often perceived as a cosmetic cure-alls, IPL, excimer lasers, and the Fraxel Restore laser are the only light-based procedures that have been suggested by the doctors on RealSelf for hypopigmentation treatment. For patients who experience extreme hypopigmentation on over half of their body (a rare occurrence of vitiligo), overall depigmentation is a option.

✓ **Topical medications**: topical agents such as hydroquinone, Retinol, and other skin lightening agents, may be used to bleach skin not affected by hypopigmentation so that it can blend in better with hypopigmented skin. For hypopigmentation that is unresponsive to medications, camouflaging with cosmetic tattooing or permanent makeup may be the best option.

Knowing qualified and experienced Aesthetician or doctors are the first step for successful removal of dark spots and abnormal pigmentation. Professional experts will study your condition, look at your case and then suggest a treatment tailor-made for your pigmentation problem. You can always Contact me to receive the most effective anti-aging treatment.

17

<u>Chapter 2</u>

Pigmentation Reasons

Have you ever wondered why you still get pigmentation on your skin even though you've been avoiding the sun like a plague? Perhaps you're thinking your sunscreen is useless? Well, while excessive exposure to sunlight is one of the main causes for dark spots on the skin, Irregular areas in which there are changes to skin colour are much more common than you might think. Often, you may have changes in the pigmentation of a certain area of your skin due to a difference in the level of melanin it contains. Melanin is the substance that provides colour to the skin and protects it from the sun. However, there are a wide range of reasons and causes that can contribute to skin pigmentation you may not be aware ofsome of which are listed below:

20 Pigmentation Triggers

1. **Stress** - If you thought your stress has no effect on your skin, you are mistaken. When you are stressed out, the free radicals in your body increase in number. This can

aggravate skin pigmentation and also give rise to new spots.

2. **Sun exposure** - One of the worst causes of skin pigmentation, sun exposure increases this further if you do not take adequate protection. Always applies a sunscreen lotion of at least 30 SPF before stepping out and reapplies it every two hours. Even if it is cloudy, make sure you have it on as the rays can still penetrate your skin.

3. **Perfumed products** - How we love products that have a good fragrance. But these can lead to skin pigmentation as well. If you have sensitive skin or a history of allergies, you should definitely avoid using products that are perfumed. Also, do not spray perfumes directly on your skin.

4. **Hormonal imbalance** - When there is a hormonal imbalance in your body, you are likely to suffer from skin pigmentation. This could also be a symptom of an underlying condition such as thyroid disorder, kidney and liver disease, insulin resistance, etc. It is essential to address this problem and get yourself checked by a doctor.

5. **Heat from sauna and cooking** - It's not only the scorching sun that'll give you pigmentation. Heat from fire, cooking and sauna are culprits too, basically anything that

stimulates the pigment cells. According to Dermatologist Cheryl Lee Eberting, heat can worsen one's melasma. Dermatologic Surgeon Sabrina Fabi also indicated that a study they did that skin browning was intimately associated with underlying blood vessels that dilate and get worse with heat. Anything that causes excess heat can lead to pigmentation. If your skin is prone to it, you may want to avoid cooking on high flame as it can produce intense heat. If this is unavoidable, apply a protective cream on areas exposed before you cook. Also, avoid using the sauna, the steam room, or doing hot yoga.

6. **Poor blood circulation** - Poor blood circulation often results in a lack of oxygen in the blood and hence, this can also cause skin pigmentation, dark spots or blotchy complexion. Logically, an improved blood circulation could prevent this.

7. **Lack of sleep** - Lack of sleep is a major contributor to pigmentation because it can wreak havoc at different levels. One, it causes poor blood circulation and this results in a lack of oxygen in the blood and hence, this can also cause skin pigmentation, dark spots or blotchy complexion. Next, sleep deprivation can increase stress hormones that causes skin pigmentation. One such

hormone I read is the adrenocorticotropic hormone, which causes an increase in skin pigmentation. And according to a report published at NCBI, adrenocorticotropic hormone released by stress may activate tyrosinase in melanocytes, resulting in the augmentation of ultraviolet-induced pigmentation.

8. **Hormonal changes** - Abnormal levels in estrogen and progesterone are major culprits of pigmentation. Heard of melasma? This may be caused by taking birth control pills, pregnancy, and illnesses. Even some foods can cause this problem. Examples include soy, and flax which are packed with estrogen. I found out that excessive consumption of coffee as well as food microwaved in plastic containers are contributors too.

9. **Smoking** - Smoking not only exposes your body and skin to several toxic chemicals, it also reduces antioxidants which are responsible for renewing and keeping your skin healthy. These two factors can cause skin pigmentation.

10. **Using bad skincare products** - You may be cleansing and toning your skin every day but if your skincare products are of poor quality, you are likely to have skin pigmentation. It is vital to use products that are natural

and suit your skin well. Always search for user reviews if you aren't sure if the company is good or not.

11. **Hair colouring** - Just like bleaching leads to skin pigmentation, even colouring your hair as the same effect. This is because even though you are coloring your hair, the chemicals present in it can be passed on your skin as well. So avoid doing this or opt for chemical-free, natural hair colors. Avoid ones that have harsh chemicals in them.

12. **Friction** - When their is friction, there are chances of skin pigmentation. It can be easily created by the use of nylon loofahs or by scrubbing your skin vigorously. It can also dry out your skin and make it flaky.

13. **Acne** - Some of you may have realized by now that your acne marks can become a permanent pigmented spot. This is referred to as post-inflammatory hyperpigmentation, which appears as flat spots of discolouration. Besides acne, other causes for post-inflammatory hyperpigmentation include atopic dermatitis or psoriasis. Even injuries caused by dermabrasion, chemical peels or laser-therapies can trigger skin pigmentation. While all skin types can get post-inflammatory hyperpigmentation, it is more prevalent in darker tones of skin.

14. **Parabens** - Many readings suggest that parabens are estrogenic but what caught my attention was that studies indicate that methylparaben applied on the skin reacts with UVB leading to increase skin aging and DNA damage. These results indicate that methylparaben may have harmful effects on human skin when exposed to sunlight. I'll probably get a lot of flaks for this but do note that I am citing a credible study. You can say the results are inconclusive and speculative but that makes any refute against it equally inconclusive and speculative.

15. **Menstruation cycle** - Not only is our skin vulnerable to UV radiation during PMS, we should avoid sun exposure as far as possible one week prior to our menses to avoid developing skin pigmentation. This is because our female hormonal activity of estrogen and/or progesterone is causing melanocytes or the pigment-producing cells to produce and deposit excess pigments. Interestingly, I found a study that supports that the skin of women is more sensitive to ultra-violent light in the premenstrual week. From the study, about half the women questioned had some increase in skin pigmentation, which was noted in every case in the latter days of the menstrual cycle and in some cases during menstruation also.

16. **Cosmetics laden with heavy metals** - Heavy metals produce increased pigmentation in part from deposition of metal particles and in part from an increase in epidermal melanin production. The antimalarials may bind to melanin. Lead, bismuth, mercury, silver, arsenic, and gold.

17. **Infections** - Infections are a common reason for localized changes in skin color. Cuts and scrapes regularly develop infections that turn the surrounding skin red or white and change the texture too. Erythrasma, Tinea versicolor, and ringworm are all infections that can cause patches of skin to turn white, pink, tan, or brown and scaly. The patches can occur all over the body, depending on the exact type of fungus.

18. **Skin cancer** - Cancer can change skin colour or texture. Your doctor should examine moles or other rapidly changing skin lesions.

19. **Birthmarks** - Birthmarks are also a cause of skin colour changes.

Café-au-lait spots are light-coloured spots on the skin. Few café-au-lait spots are perfectly normal, but more than six may be an indicator of neurofibromatosis, a genetic disorder that negatively affects the growth and formation of nerve cells.

Moles are brown spots that can appear on the skin at birth. Changes in the size or shape of these spots can signal trouble, and should be checked by your doctor.

Mongolian blue spots are bluish patches that can appear on the backs of babies and young children, usually of Asian descent. They are harmless and often fade over time.

Port-wine stains are a type of birthmark caused by swollen blood vessels. They are usually flat and appear pink or red in colour.

20. **Autoimmune diseases and allergies** - Autoimmune diseases, such as lupus erythematosus and dermatomyositis, can be responsible for changes in skin color, whilst Eczema is a type of hypersensitivity reaction (allergy) that can cause red, scaly patches that ooze. Related to eczema, pityriasis alba can cause dry, white patches on the skin in children. A wide variety of rashes, such as dermatitis herpetiform, contact dermatitis, poison ivy rashes, and others can be caused by a allergic reaction. Scleroderma can create thick, shiny patches of skin. Vitiligo is a condition in which cells that produce melanin are attacked by the immune system, leavingbehind patches of skin with no color at all.

Chapter 3

Determine Your Skin Color

Human Skin Color

Your complexion is a unique reflection of your ethnicity, race, genetics, and exposures, and beauty certainly comes in all shades. Moreover, traditional labels like "black" and "white" do not appropriately capture how skin tone varies among individuals. After all, there are "black" people with pale white skin, and "white" people with dark brown skin.

Human skin color ranges in variety from the darkest brown to the lightest hues. An individual's skin pigmentation is the result of genetics, being the product of both of the individual's biological parents' genetic makeup. In evolution, skin pigmentation in human beings evolved by a process of natural selection primarily to regulate the amount of ultraviolet radiation penetrating the skin, controlling its biochemical effects.

The actual skin color of different humans is affected by many substances, although the single most important substance is the pigment melanin. Melanin is produced within the skin in cells called melanocytes and it is the main determinant of the skin color of darker-skinned humans. The skin color of people with light skin is determined mainly by the bluish-white connective tissue under the dermis and by the hemoglobin circulating in the veins of the dermis. The red color underlying the skin becomes more visible, especially in the face, when, as consequence of physical exercise or the stimulation of the nervous system (anger, fear). Color is not entirely uniform across an individual's skin; for example, the skin of the palm and the sole is lighter than most other skin, and this is especially noticeable in darker-skinned people.

There is a direct correlation between the geographic distribution of UV radiation (UVR) and the distribution of indigenous skin pigmentation around the world. Areas that receive higher amounts of UVR, generally located closer to the equator, tend to have darker-skinned populations. Areas that are far from the tropics and closer to the poles have lower intensity of UVR, which is reflected in lighter-skinned populations. Researchers suggests that human populations over the past 50,000 years have changed from dark-skinned to light-skinned and vice versa as they migrated to different UV zones, and that such major changes in pigmentation may have happened in as little as 100 generations ($\approx$2,500 years) through selective sweeps. Natural skin color can also darken as a result of tanning due to exposure to sunlight. The leading theory is that skin color adapts to intense sunlight irradiation to provide partial protection against the ultraviolet fraction that produces damage and thus mutations in the DNA of the skin cells.Besides, it has been observed that adult human females on average are significantly lighter in skin pigmentation than males. Females need more calcium during pregnancy and lactation. The body synthesizes vitamin D from sunlight, which helps it absorb calcium. Females evolved to have lighter skin so their bodies absorb more calcium.The social significance of differences in skin color has varied across cultures and over time, as demonstrated with regard to social status and discrimination.

Melanin And Genes

Melanin is produced by cells called melanocytes in a process called melanogenesis. Melanin is made within small membrane–bound packages called melanosomes. As they become full of melanin, they move into the slender arms of melanocytes, from where they are transferred to the keratinocytes. Under normal conditions, melanosomes cover the upper part of the keratinocytes and protect them from genetic damage. One melanocyte supplies melanin to thirty-six keratinocytes according to signals from the keratinocytes. They also regulate melanin production and replication of melanocytes.People have different skin colors mainly because of their melanocytes produce different amount and kinds of melanin.

The genetic mechanism behind human skin color is mainly regulated by the enzyme tyrosinase, which creates the color of the skin, eyes, and hair shades.Differences in skin color are also attributed to differences in size and distribution of melanosomes in the skin. Melanocytes produce two types of melanin. The most common form of biological melanin is eumelanin, a brown-black polymer of dihydroxyindole carboxylic acids, and their reduced forms. Most is derived from the amino acid tyrosine. Eumelanin is found in hair, areola, and skin, and the hair colors gray, black, blond, and brown. In humans, it is more abundant in people with dark skin. Pheomelanin, a pink to red hue is found in particularly large quantities in red hair,the lips, nipples, glans of the penis, and vagina.

Both the amount and type of melanin produced is controlled by a number of genes that operate under incomplete dominance.One copy of each of the various genes is inherited from each parent. Each gene can come in several alleles, resulting in the great variety of human skin tones. Melanin controls the amount of ultraviolet (UV) radiation from the sun that penetrates the skin by absorption. While UV radiation can assist in the production of vitamin D, excessive exposure to UV can damage health.

Fitzpatrick Skin Types

If you've ever tried to match foundation or concealer to your skin, you know just how tricky skin typing can be. Fitzpatrick skin typing is a scientific skin type classification. Though, this form of skin typing, won't help you find your perfect shade, it can tell you just how much shade you should get on sunny days.

Developed in 1975, the system classifies skin type according to the amount of pigment your skin has and your skin's reaction to sun exposure. This information can help predict your overall risk of sun damage and skin cancer. Once you know your risk level, you can arm yourself with the tools you need to protect your skin.

The Six Skin Types

This classification is semi-subjective, as it was developed by interviewing people about their past sun reactions. After picking out distinct trends, the creator identified six groups. It's possible that you won't meet all of the characteristics of any one type, so you should go with the one that best describes you.

Fitzpatrick skin type 1

- ✓ skin color (before sun exposure): ivory

- ✓ eye color: light blue, light gray, or light green

- ✓ natural hair color: red or light blonde

- ✓ sun reaction: skin always freckles, always burns and peels, and never tans

Fitzpatrick skin type 2

- ✓ Skin color (before sun exposure): fair or pale

- ✓ Eye color: blue, gray, or green

- ✓ natural hair color: blonde

- ✓ sun reaction: skin usually freckles, burns and peels often, and rarely tans

Fitzpatrick skin type 3

- ✓ Skin color (before sun exposure): fair to beige, with golden undertones

- ✓ Eye color: hazel or light brown

- ✓ Natural hair color: dark blonde or light brown

✓ Sun reaction: skin might freckle, burns on occasion, and sometimes tans

Fitzpatrick skin type 4

✓ Skin color (before sun exposure): olive or light brown

✓ Eye color: dark brown

✓ Natural hair color: dark brown

✓ Sun reaction: doesn't really freckle, burns rarely, and tans often

Fitzpatrick skin type 5

✓ Skin color (before sun exposure): dark brown or black

✓ Eye color: dark brown to black

✓ Natural hair color: dark brown to black

✓ Sun reaction: rarely freckles, almost never burns, and always tans

Fitzpatrick skin type 6

✓ Skin color (before sun exposure): black

✓ Eye color: brownish black

✓ Natural hair color: black

✓ Sun reaction: never freckles, never burns, and always tans darkly

Skin Type Treatment

Tanning beds and other artificial tanning machines are harmful for everyone, regardless of skin type. Some research suggests that people who use tanning machines before age 35 years are 75 times more likely to develop melanoma in their lifetime.

Your risk of sun damage is also higher if you live near the equator. The closer to the equator you are, the more intense the sun's rays are, so being vigilant about sun protection is crucial. Everyone should apply sunscreen daily to receive maximum protection. Here's what else you should know about your skin and how to protect it based on your skin type.

Types 1 and 2

If your skin type is 1 or 2, you have a high risk of:

- sun damage

- skin aging from sun exposure

- melanoma and other skin cancers

You should follow these tips to protect your skin:

- Use a sunscreen with an SPF of 30 or higher.

- Limit your sun exposure and seek shade whenever you're out in the sun.

- Wear an hat with a wide brim to protect your head and face.

- Wear UV-blocking sunglasses.

- Wear protective clothing with a UPF rating of 30 or higher if you plan to be in direct sunlight for extended periods.

- Check your skin from head to toe each month.

- Have an annual skin checkup with a doctor.

Types 3 to 6

If your skin is type 3 to 6, you still have some risk of skin cancer from sun exposure, especially if you've used an indoor tanning bed. You should always use sun protection even though your risk is lower than people's with type 1 or 2 skin.

The Skin Cancer Foundation notes that African-Americans who have been diagnosed with melanoma usually are often diagnosed at a later stage, contributing to a poorer overall outlook.

For maximum protection, you should follow these tips:

- Limit your sun exposure.

- Wear an hat with a wide brim to protect your head and face.

- Wear UV-blocking sunglasses.

- Wear protective clothing if you plan to be in direct sunlight for extended periods.

- Wear sunscreen with an SPF of 15 or higher.

- Check your skin from head to toe each month. Pay careful attention to any strange growths. Acral lentiginous melanoma is the dominant form of melanoma among darker-skinned people. It appears on parts of the body not often exposed to the sun. It's usually undetected until after the cancer has spread, so make sure you check all areas of your body.

- Have an annual skin checkup with a doctor.

When to get screened

If you're at an increased risk of skin cancer, you should have regular skin exams. Talk to your doctor about how often you should come in for a screening. Depending on your individual needs, skin screening could be more frequent than your annual checkup.

People at increased risk of skin cancer include those who have:

- personal or family history of skin cancer

- Fitzpatrick skin type 1 or 2

- a compromised immune system

It's important to be aware of any change in skin discoloration and consult your doctor with any change. Using whitening creams day and night will definitely reduce your risk for skin pigmentation and problems.

<u>Chapter 4</u>

Pigmentation Treatment

Firstly, don't panic! There are a number of ways to treat your pigmentation changes, from great make up, to microdermabrasion or topical bleaching creams. Diagnosis of the reason behind your pigmentation changes is key though, as not all 'dark spots' are created equal.One of the best ways to avoid pigmentation is to fastidiously applying a sunscreen with a minimum SPF of 30+, which will block both UVA and UVB light. The sunscreen needs to be applied every three to four hours if you're outdoors. If you're unsure or worried, then make an appointment to see your doctor before attempting any drastic treatments. Below we look at hyper and hypopigmentation in more detail.

Whitening Creams

A skin bleaching cream can be used to visibly reduce the appearance of sun damage, age spots, freckles, acne marks, old scars, birthmarks, melasma and uneven skin tones.

A skin bleaching cream works in two different ways:

- Absorbing the UV rays preventing the sun from darkening your skin

- Reducing the production of melanin, the pigment responsible for skin darkening

Most skin bleaching creams contain ingredients that can reduce the amount of melanin production by inhibiting tyrosinase, a key enzyme to melanin synthesis.

A bleaching or whitening cream is not a product you should buy in a rush. You need to choose wisely and carefully, because of some skin bleaching creams may contain ingredients with serious side skin effects. The first thing to do before buying a skin bleaching cream is to check the ingredients it contains. This will allow you to discard the creams that contain chemicals that can be harmful or that are banned.

REMEMBER: if your skin is in the 1-3 numbers of Fitzpatrick you can start with the medium strength of creams, but if your skin is from 3-6 you should start with a low concentration of Retinol and Alpha Acids for a long time before using the strong grade creams.

For any skin type, the key is to start using lightening creams gradually, start with mild AHA and BHA acids in the morning and mild retinol cream (1% and less) in the evening and continue to stronger creams preferably professional cream.

The Must Ingredients:

When you buy an Anti-Pigmentation cream look for the following ingredients that will get an active treatment for your face:

Retinol (vitamin A) -Vitamin A is a powerful antioxidant that neutralizes free radicals that cause premature aging usually (Free radicals break down skin cells and collagen in the skin). It reduces the appearance and depth of wrinkles, and It stimulates the cellular renewal of the skin. Retinol is also known as vitamin A, retinoic acid and retinoid. Retinol is widely used to treat severe acne and rosacea. Retinoids reduce wrinkles, freckles, blackheads, and stains caused by sunlight. It takes about 3 months for the skin acclimates to a retinoid.

A/B-hydroxy acids (AHA or BHA) - AHA and BHA are widely used in the cosmetic industry because they remove the top layer of dead skin cells and stimulate the growth of healthy new cells. A-hydroxy acids work as exfoliating agents, they have a cooling effect on the skin and improve its overall appearance.

A-hydroxy acids penetrate deep into the dermis and stimulate the production of collagen and elastin fibers which are essential for healthy skin. A-hydroxy acids generally used include: glycolic acid, lactic acid and salicylic acid. You should know that all types of α-hydroxy acids increase susceptibility to the harmful effects of the sun and it is essential to use sunscreen daily to avoid sun damage.

Hydroquinone -Hydroquinone is used as a topical application in skin whitening to reduce the color of skin. It does not have the same predisposition to cause dermatitis as metal does. This is a prescription only ingredient in some countries, including the member states of the European Union. While using hydroquinone as a lightening agent can be effective with proper use, it can also cause skin sensitivity. Using a daily sunscreen with a high PPD (persistent pigment darkening) rating reduces the risk of further damage. Hydroquinone is sometimes combined with alpha hydroxy acids that exfoliate the skin to quicken the lightening process. In the United States, topical treatments usually contain up to 2% in hydroquinone. Otherwise, higher concentrations (up to 4%) should be prescribed and used with caution.

Peptides -Peptides penetrates the outer layer of the skin and repair. Some Peptides can inhibit the production of melanin in the skin like copper peptides and the best peptide named Epidermosil that works like retinol but is not dangerous in the sun so you can use it in the morning to prevent sun damage.

Vitamin C -Vitamin C is an antioxidant with a brightening effect of the skin. It is a common component in products for skin care as well as makeup products because it gives the skin a youthful and stimulates blood circulation. Vitamin C also keeps the skin elastic and prevents premature aging. When combined with vitamin E it reduces the signs of aging: wrinkles, fine lines, brown spots and age spots. Vitamin C is also known as ascorbic acid.

Vitamin E -Vitamin E provides natural protection against harmful UV rays, Vitamin E creates a moisture barrier and prevents the discoloration of the skin. It helps the skin to repair itself.

Antioxidants - The most common are vitamin A, vitamin C and vitamin E. Antioxidants neutralize free radicals and prevent premature aging of the skin. Many beauty products like cleansers, moisturizing lotions, tonics, claim to contain antioxidants.

Glutathione Skin Whitening

Glutathione is the body's most potent and vital antioxidants, present in every cell in the body. It plays a pivotal role in detoxifying our cells, removing heavy metals, toxins, and free radicals. All of which can damage our cells and significantly damage the quality of our cells, including skin cells.

Age spots can also be minimized and prevented by enhancing Glutathione levels in the body. The anti-aging effects of Glutathione are remarkable, from complexion, age spots and wrinkles, there is very little that won't benefit from this master antioxidant.

Glutathione pills help to whiten the skin in a couple of different ways. I would not recommend injecting Glutathione by yourself or any expert or doctor, this injection is not considered safe and has some side effects. Melanin is the pigment that gives our skin its color, produced by the activation of the enzyme Tyrosinase. GSH binds to Tyrosinase and helps prevent the enzymatic pathways from producing melanin. The second is a much more important role. GSH helps to prevent the activation of Tyrosinase by reducing free radicals in the body that can activate it and cause an increase in melanin production.

There are plenty of glutathione creams on the market and many of which are quality. Just like supplementation, it's all a matter of doing your research.The pitfall of Glutathione creams is the fact that we don't get the full benefit of this fantastic antioxidant. By supplementing with L-glutathione or acetyl glutathione, you are harnessing the full potential of this Master Antioxidant. Fight aging from the source, improve the health of your cells and improve the look of your skin. All while you help prevent disease, increase your energy levels; helping you look and feel younger.

Do not expect dramatic results within a few weeks of supplementing Glutathione. What you can expect is healthier skin, hair, and nails by supplementing with a top quality Glutathione supplement regularly. Ridding your body of harmful toxins and optimizing your cellular health.

It is best to think of a Glutathione as a total body health supplement that has skin health benefits, one of which being improved skin pigmentation. It is far more than just a skin whitener; it is the single most important antioxidant for your overall health and well-being.

Pigmentation Secret

The Big Pigmentation Secret - Treating the skin from the inside and making cell circulation is the secret for treating pigmentation. It is usually called Mesotherapy. Meso means middle And therapy - is a treatment. Which means that the method takes care of the middle of the skin, deep within the dermis. This technique, which began to develop in 1952, is a penetrating therapeutic and Natural active ingredients into the subcutaneous skin thus effectively treat the skin. Use of natural ingredients is highly recommended and is an inseparable part of the treatment of mesotherapy because the nutrients are absorbed into the skin and flow into the bloodstream.

Because the skin-applied substances remain in the area for a long time, this method is excellent for treating pigmentation of all sorts and kinds mentioned above.

Using a skin care roller is one of the most effective ways to get flawless skin.

The use of the roller has been known for more than 4000 years and has been developed in China as part of the acupuncture method that acts on the meridian points in the body and activates the energy of the chi, which is the energy of life in the treated area.

The use of a roller for the long-term causes the skin to be generally less sensitive to skin problems such as seborrhea, psoriasis, acne and sensitized or irritated skin.

Professional Home Treatment

The most powerful treatment is one that you can DIY with a simple home Roller. Roller with needles in different sizes according to the type of roller actually activates three mechanisms associated with anti-aging.

1. Renew - Smoothing the Roller needles on the skin actually causes a controlled skin injury. This process produces mechanical exfoliation that helps to clear melanin and dead skin cells in all treated areas.

2. Nourish -The roller opens microscopic holes in the skin At a depth of 0.3-2 mm (depending on the type of roller you use), and therefore all the products you use after the treatment penetrate to the depth of the skin, and you get up to thirty times more activity from the cosmetics products you use.

3. Repair -The mechanism of the wound itself, although this is a microscopic injury but the skin works to repair itself. This process helps to rebuild the area treated with collagen and elastin, which are the basic building blocks of the skin, which flow from the body and contribute to the building and solidification of the treated area. Significant results can be achieved by multiple Treatment for Pigmentation, wrinkles, scars, and sores for all skin types, suitable for use at any age, easy to operate and gives cumulative results over time.

The Roller is the most effective tool known for science and cosmetic research. It is the cheapest treatment you can do to yourself in the comfort of your home with great results even compared to laser or IPL treatments. I suggest that you use the Roller at least once a week, on one regular day to maximize skin care efficiency.

Effective Pigmentation Treatment

If creams do not work, chemical peels, microdermabrasion or fractional lasers are further treatment options. These procedures require multiple sessions at intervals of one to four weeks.

Microdermabrasion

The SkinBase microdermabrasion facial was designed as a skin pigmentation treatment and can therefore vastly improve the appearance of facial pigmentation and skin blemishes, especially melasma. Microdermabrasion will ultimately act as a treatment for your pigmentation, gently removing a layer of skin and removing the dark skin which has formed. The final result and the number of treatments depend on on a number of factors including the type of lesion, skin type, the degree of suntan,

size and depth of the vessels and the location to be treated. Your SkinBase therapist will advise you on the number of treatments during your consultation session.

Remember, it is even more important than ever to protect your skin with a high factor sun cream following microdermabrasion due to the crystals gently buffing away the dead skins that may have been helping to protect your skin.

AHA (Glycolic Acid) and BHA (Salicylic Acid) Peels

Light chemical peels contain alpha hydroxy acids and beta hydroxy acids are a great way to eliminate pigmentation. Aestheticians and Physicians who perform light chemical peels select a appropriatechemical solution(or mix of solutions) based on each patient's needs. Chemical peels primarily containing alpha hydroxy acids may be referred to as "AHA chemical peels" or "glycolic acid peels." Glycolic acid is the most common type of alpha hydroxy acid used in skin care. Salicylic acid chemical peels are the most common type of beta hydroxy acid peel.

Alpha hydroxy acids (AHAs) are derived from fruit, sugar, sour milk, and other natural sources.

AHA chemical peels often contain:

- ✓ Glycolic acid (extracted from sugar cane)

- ✓ Lactic acid (extracted from milk)

- ✓ Malic acid (extracted from pears and apples)

- ✓ Citric acid (extracted from oranges and lemons)

- ✓ Tartaric acid (extracted from grapes)

Beta hydroxy acids are simple organic acids derived from fruit. When a physician refers to " salicylic acid chemical peels," he or she is referring to a beta hydroxy acid. Though closely related to alpha hydroxy acids, beta hydroxy acids differ slightly in their molecular structure, and rejuvenate the skin in a slightly different way. The most common beta hydroxy acid, salicylic acid, has been used for decades as an acne remedy, and salicylic acid chemical peels are especially effective in eliminating acne. Beta hydroxy acids are helpful because they can exfoliate oily skin and deeply penetrate the skin with no irritation.

Regardless of the specific type, Alpha hydroxy and beta hydroxy acids gently rejuvenate the skin and encourage skin cell regeneration with little or no irritation or discomfort. Glycolic acid, salicylic acid, lactic acid, and other alpha hydroxy acids are so gentle, in fact, that they are common ingredients in home skin care products, and patients who undergo a light chemical peel may be asked to use such products to improve on their results.

Make Up For Flawless Skin

Suddenly noticing the appearance of dark spots or pigmentation can be a real blow to your confidence, but as with many flaws – a great make up technique can be your saviour.

Chapter 5

Avoid Pigmentation

Pigmentation spots are characterized by brown, black or sometimes red spots that appear on the surface of the skin. More often than not, these spots are caused by too much sun exposure. One of the best ways to avoid pigmentation is to fastidiously apply a sunscreen with a minimum SPF of 30+, which will block both UVA and UVB light. The sunscreen needs to be applied every three to four hours if you're outdoors. Topical creams containing hydroquinone, retinol, alpha hydroxy acid creams, azelic acid or kojic acid should be used at nightime together with sunblock during the day. Oral use of antioxidants also help in reducing pigmentation. If creams do not work, chemical peels, microdermabrasion or fractional lasers are further treatment options. These procedures require multiple sessions at intervals of one to four weeks.

The UV rays of the sun trigger a abnormal melanin production in the skin. This often happens to people with fairer skin. In addition to sun exposure, these spots can also form because of damages to the surface layer of the dermis. When you scratch or bump your dry dermis, it can get easily wounded. Find out today how you can prevent these spots from forming:

The To Do List

1. Use a lightening moisturizer daily - There are many people who will cringe at the idea of using lightening moisturizers. This product is actually a little tricky to use. If you are not using an appropriate one, it can lead to disastrous results. This is why you should go look for a product that contains more natural ingredients. Chemical products will make your skin photosensitive when you go out in the sun. You will get later on all the information you need about lightening and whitening creams.

2. Maintain skin health by using face mask regularly - Avocado and Lemon are ideal ingredients in making face skin mask. This can help repair the damages brought about by prolonged sun exposure. This can also help reduce the appearance of sun or age spots. You can add a bit of honey in the mask and apply it on your skin. Leave the mask there for at least one hour before washing it off. If you do not have avocado, papaya is a good substitute.

3. Scrub your skin every day - The surface layer of your dermis is cluttered with toxins, bacteria, sebum, dead skin cells and much more unwanted stuff. If you do not get rid of them, the moisturizing creams you are using will not penetrate deeper. Use a gentle scrub such as rice, sugar and lemon juice. This will clean your skin deep down.

4. Sun And Skin - We all know we need to protect our skin from the sun's harmful rays. Of course, it's impossible to avoid the sun. who wants to hide indoors when it feels so great to get outside? And the sun's not all bad, anyway: Sunlight helps our bodies create vitamin D. So follow these tips when you're outdoors to help manage sun exposure:

- Wear sunscreen with a sun protection factor (SPF) of at least 30, even if it's cloudy or you don't plan on spending a lot of time outdoors. If you sweat a lot or go swimming, reapply sunscreen every 1½ to 2 hours (even if the bottle says the sunscreen is waterproof).

- Choose a sunscreen that blocks both UVA and UVB rays. Look for the words "broad spectrum protection" or UVA protection in addition to the SPF of 30 or greater. Select a sunscreen that says "nonacnegenic" or "noncomedogenic" on the label to help keep pores clear.

- The sun's rays are strongest between 10 a.m. and 4 p.m., so reapply sunscreen frequently and take breaks indoors if you can. If your shadow is longer than you are tall, then it's a safer time to be in the sun (you should still wear sunscreen, though).

- Apply more sunscreen (with 30 and higher SPF) when you're around reflective surfaces like water, snow, or ice.

- We all know that the sun can damage skin, but did you know it can contribute to eye problems, too? Protect your face and eyes with a hat and sunglasses that provide 100% UV protection.

- Some medications, such as prescription acne medications, can increase your sensitivity to the sun (and to tanning beds). So if you're taking medication, increase your sun protection.

- If you want the glow of a tan, try faking it with self-tanners. Avoid tanning beds. They still contain some of the same harmful UV rays as the sun.

Long Run Treatment

Treating pigmentation is a life taking process. People who tend to pigmentation and want to have spotless skin must use lightening cream for life as the regular skincare regime. The sooner you understand how important it is to take care of your skin to maintain a feeling of youth and vitality, the better it is. A skin care regimen needs to be developed early in the teen years and should be carried on so that you can ensure that your skin remain plump, keeps glowing and looks beautiful as you age.

You needs to cleanse and nourish your skin on a daily basis, and all the marketers out there know that they also know that you will buy anything that comes your way if it promises you youthful skin in few minutes. It is important that you to learn to identify the good from the bad and only choose skin care products that are natural and suit your skin type and are not ridden with chemicals that are only going to do your skin harm in the long run.

Remember - Even when the spots are removed with a laser or peel if the skin is not treated with lightening creams all the pigmentation will come back and the treatment will be worthless.

Chapter 6

Home Remedies

Natural Pigmentation Treatments

Natural treatment of the face and body is vital. Treating pigmentation naturally should include all your cosmetic needs. You can get my free recipe book offer and start treating yourself with respect to nature; you can prepare at home anything or product your body needs.

Melasma - This is a skin pigmentation disorder that appears on the face in the form of tan or brown patches, especially the forehead, cheeks, upper lip, nose, and chin. Melasma is typically seen in pregnant women. The spots generally fade after pregnancy, but sometimes they just don't go away. It may also occur in women on birth control pills or postmenopausal estrogen. Well, men, too can get melasma sometimes. Some Ayurvedic practitioners believe that this disorder can also be caused by nutritional deficiencies, so that can explain why men too might get melasma.

Home Remedies for Melasma:

Orange Paste: Grate the skin of an orange and make a paste / gel with few teaspoons of milk. Leave it on for half an hour and then massage gently and wash it off with warm water. Exfoliate your face at least 3 to 4 times a week with this paste. Exfoliation encourages cell renewal and removes the dark blotches.

Aloe Vera Juice to Lighten Dark Spots: Gently applies aloe vera juice or gel on the affected area and leave it on for 15 minutes. Wash it off with warm water. Aloe vera contains mucilaginous polysaccharides that can effectively lighten dark spots.

Turmeric Powder and Milk: Make a paste of 5 tablespoons of turmeric powder in 10 tablespoons of milk and apply it all over your face. Gently massage your face and wash it off with warm water after 20 minutes.

Almond and Honey Face Pack: Make a face pack with almond and honey. Apply and wash it off after 15 minutes.

Triphala Choornam: Ayurvedic practitioners recommend taking 1 tablespoon of Triphala Choornam with warm water at bed time to accelerate healing.

Use Sunscreen: Sunlight worsens the condition, so use sunscreen at all times.

Vitiligo - Vitiligo It is a disorder where the immune system of the body attacks the pigment cells, and the consequent loss of pigments causes smooth, white skin patches, usually around the mouth and eyes, or on the back of the hands. In some people, the skin discoloration can appear all over the body. Vitiligo can also occur if you suffer from the disease associated with immune system disorder such as diabetes, pernicious anemia, thyroid disease, or Addison's disease. Although there is actually no cure for this disorder, certain home remedies can help treat the condition, but it may take a long time before you can see the difference.

Home Remedies for Vitiligo:

Foods to Avoids: It is best to avoid sour foods including sour fruit juices, This is because sour foods shift the pH balance of the body to acidic, but for melanin production, you need a more alkaline base. Avoid sea food too because of contaminants such as mercury.

Keep Hydrated: Drinking water kept overnight in a copper vessel can help reduce vitiligo patches. Make it a habit.

Turmeric and Mustard Oil Paste: Prepare a mixture of 5 teaspoons of turmeric powder in 250 ml of mustard oil. Apply the paste twice daily to the affected area. It may take up to a year to see the results.

Bakuchi and Coconut Oil Mix: Powder the seeds of Bakuchi (Psoralea coryifolia), mix it in coconut oil. Apply to the affected area. Not exactly a home remedy, but you can buy Bakuchi oil straight away and use it topically for vitiligo for more effectiveness.

Bakuchi and Tamarind Seeds: Soak Bakuchi seeds and tamarind seeds in the water you washed the rice grains with and keep it for a week. Grind it to a paste and apply to the leukoderma patches. It is said to give quick results.

Ginger Juice: Apply a mixture of ginger juice and red clay to the affected area. It might take a long time to heal, but it is effective.

Radish Seeds and Vinegar: Mix 25g of the powdered white radish seeds and two teaspoon of vinegar. Apply it over the patches daily. This is also a long treatment.

Post Inflammatory Hyperpigmentation or Hypopigmentation

Home Remedies for Hyper/Hypopigmentation:

The Power Of Potato Treatment: Potatoes are not just good sources of starch but can also prevent a host of skin pigmentation problems like melasma, dark circles, hyper and hypo pigmentation. Potatoes can lighten the skin with continuous application. For using potatoes for pigmentation, slice one medium sized potato into two and put few drops of water on the surface. Rub it on the pigmented area so that the juice of potato acts on the skin. If you have more time at hand, grate the potatoes and squeeze the juice out of it. Apply on the age spots and leave it on for half an hour. Rinse with warm water. Doing this for a month will present you with noticeable difference in your pigmented skin.

Almonds, Cream and Lemon Juice Pack: Make a paste with 5 almonds, fresh cream and few drops of lemon juice. Apply to the affected area and leave it on for 15 minutes. Wash it off with water.

Skin Pigmentation Removal

Lemon And Cucumber: Two wonderful skin lightening agents when put together can surely work wonders. The cool caress of cucumber and the lightening action of lemon do not disappoint, provided you give it enough importance and apply it every day. Apply every day in the morning and evening and leave it on for 20 minutes.If you do not have both these lightening agents, do not worry. They can create wonderful results when applied on their own as well. Lemon is a natural bleach and cucumber is used for dark circles which too is a form of skin pigmentation.

Papaya Face Pack to Remove Sun Tan: Apply a face mask of mashed papaya or use papaya juice on the affected area. It's a good home remedy for tans and sunburns, plus it will smoothen and improve your skin complexion.

Tomato Juice, Oatmeal and Yogurt Mix: Make a preparation of tomato juice, 2 tablespoons of oatmeal, and half a teaspoon of yogurt. Apply on the patches and rinse it off after sometime (or when it dries completely). Do it daily till you see results.

Cocoa Butter For Removing Skin Pigmentation: butter can help soothing and healing of skin due to its antioxidant properties. They protect the skin form the harsh effects of free radicals present in the atmosphere and prevent skin pigmentation by moisturising the skin. Smear cocoa butter on areas of pigmentation and massage deeply into the skin.Cocoa butter nourishes the skin and prevents the hyper pigmentation from becoming worse. Massaging improves the circulation of blood and prevents skin dryness. Both these factors are necessary for reducing and preventing hyper pigmentation.

Turmeric Powder and Lemon Juice: Add a teaspoon of lemon juice to a teaspoon of turmeric powder. Apply the paste to the affected area and leave it on for 15 minutes. Wash it off with cold water. Do not go out into the sun with the application on.

Aloe Vera Gel for Sunburn: Aloe Vera gel heals sunburn quickly. Slit opensa leaf of aloe vera and apply the gel directly to the burn. Do it 5 to 6 times daily till you see improvement.

Cornstarch Protects Against Sunburns: Another home remedy for sunburn is to dust cornstarch to the chafed areas. However, don't apply anything if the burn is blistering.

Mint Leaves to Reduces Dark Pigmentation: Grind a few mint leaves and mix it with water to form a paste. To lessen dark pigmentation, apply the paste on the melanin spots and rinse it off after 15 minutes.

Lemon Juice Cleanser: Another way to lessen hyperpigmentation is to rub a cut-half of a lemon directly to your face. If you are not comfortable with this, dilute lemon juice with water and use it as a cleanser.

Sometimes, a skin infection, blisters, tan, sunburn, other burns or other trauma to your skin, may cause a decrease or increase of pigmentation in the affected area. These pigment alterations can be reversed and home remedies work very well for such conditions.

Albinism - Albinism is an inherited disorder caused by the absence of the pigment melanin. It can occur in skin, hair, or eyes. Unfortunately, there is no cure or treatment for this in the conventional medicine, let alone a home remedy. People with albinism must use a sunscreen at all times because they are much more likely to get sun damage and skin cancer.

CONCLUSION

Because our skin is the most visible reflection of what's going on in our bodies, people equate healthy skin with beauty. But healthy skin is about more than just good looks; it's essential to our survival. So keep your skin glowing with the right skin care techniques and by eating well and getting lots of exercise.

Sunscreen will always take the first place in pigmentation treatment priorities. To avoid the most common pigmentation problems, you need to avoid excessive sun exposure and if required to go in the sun then apply a sunscreen with a minimum SPF of 30 and more. Hypo pigmented skin sunburns easily, and hyper pigmented skin may get even darker. Re apply sunscreen every two hours. Plus, to enjoy healthy skin you must follow a proper skin care routine – cleansing, toning, moisturising and exfoliating It is vitally important to remember that not one treatment will be effective on pigmentation on its own.

This is why most skin care therapists as well as doctors will recommend that you use different treatments in combination with one another. Therefore it is important to remember to use a skin care product with AHA in the morning and then cream with high levels of SPF30+, then at night use retinol cream every day.

You can consider going for IPL/Laser treatments for more efficient way of treating pigmentation than having professional creams treatments.

Take good care of the face with quality professional products and don't forget to treat the pigmentation, every week, with a Roller. Pigmentation can be beaten with good mind healthy foods and by taking good care of our faces with efficient products.

Example For Pigmentation home treatment by LAOR – day and night treatment

Laor Skin Care Series act to balance the sebaceous glands in the face and reduce the production of melanin in the skin, this action reduces skin redness and scaling that accompanies it. Amino acids, Retinol and vitamins are the most effective ingredients treating pigmentation problems. We recommend regular use of the products morning and night to keep the balance of the melanin production in the skin and thus reduce the problem of visible pigmentation.

Day Care – starts with a thorough cleansing of the skin with hydrophilic soap, product number 1 or peeling number 8. Then use cream No 21 / -21 that contain AHA and BHA. This creams balances and reduces melanin production. The daily treatment should be completed with moisture serum No 43 for extra skin whitening or moisture cream No52. It is important to put on a sun protection cream, product number 72 to reduce the effect of the sun on the skin.

Night Care – includes the removal of dead cells and dirt that has accumulated on the skin during the day, Product No 7 / 8. And in-depth of the skin treating deep melanin pigments with creams containing amino acids especially Retinol cream No 22 / -22, that helps to peel of dead cells that contribute to the accumulation of pigmentation. For best whiteningresults, it is recommended to use product No 27 that contains hydroquinone and then use serum No 42+ / 45containing a pure form of vitamin A.

It is essential to repeat here that before you launch into any of this top pigmentation treatments, consult a physician or a skin specialist. It will ensure that you choose the right treatment depending on the type of pigmentation you are suffering from, the type of skin you have and the severity of the problem.

Always remember that the pigmentation did not form overnight and it would therefore not improve overnight. It is lengthy process to lighten pigmentation; however, by following the correct methods, you will have success.

Thank you very much for reading the book. If you loved the book, I would appreciate it if you can write a review of the book for me. If you have any question about the book feel free to contact me at orilaor@outlook.com.

For 20$ Coupon for www.laorcare.com were you can find all the professional products to clear your Pigmentation, send the word: DEDICATION to my mail.

With sincere love Ori Laor

www.ingramcontent.com/pod-product-compliance
Lightning Source LLC
Chambersburg PA
CBHW060801260726
48660CB00002B/725